I0425825

This Journal Belongs To

____

www.ingramcontent.com/pod-product-compliance
Lightning Source LLC
Chambersburg PA
CBHW072058280526
45788CB00006B/2319
9781093239041